CW00520331

Published 2023

Compiled and layout design by Gary Lewis

Lewis, Gary B, 1952 —

Aging Brains … Ancient Games: keeping seniors' minds active through ancient strategy games and puzzles

1. Brain Training   2. Ancient Games and Puzzles   3. Seniors' Active Minds   I. Title

ISBN: 978-0-6455552-2-6

Digital images used and modified with permission

Published by Gary B Lewis

Cranbourne East, VICTORIA 3977

gazzablew@bigpond.com

0407219522

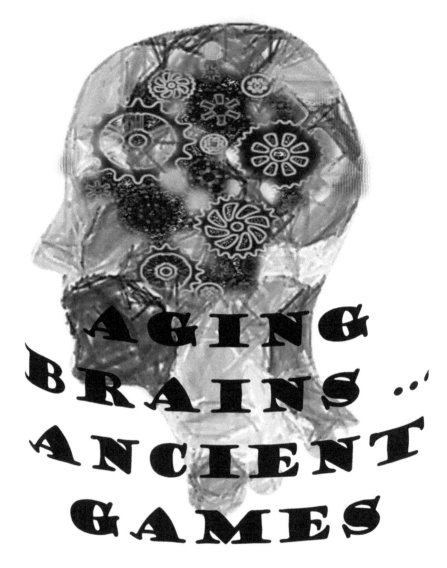

AGING BRAINS ... ANCIENT GAMES

keeping seniors' minds active through ancient strategy games

CONTENTS

BACKSTORY-FOREWORD

The games presented in this book have a proven history not only from being preserved from ancient ruin discoveries for posterity, but also from my work in education over fifty years with primary school students who embraced the simple ideas wholeheartedly.

This book offers seniors a low-cost, low-tech, option for brain training. Keeping seniors' minds alert and active is critical in an age when cognitive impairment and dementia are increasingly impacting their quality of life.

This book is designed to provide seniors an alternative to digital gaming and electronic gadgetry.

Most of these games have been salvaged and adapted from ancient traditional strategy games and puzzles — each seasoned with a modern flavour. Some games — such as Magic Squares and Arrowduko© — are simply adaptations of modern strategy games. In each chapter you will find some further backstory / historical information regarding each game as far as the author is aware.

Each game chapter will provide you with a layout, playing rules and required accessories / equipment; as well as specifying whether it is a solo activity or a two-person game.

Check out the **APPENDIX for cut-out templates**.

Let the games begin!!!

PS: The grandkids will love them too — *guaranteed!!*

SHADOWGRAMS ©

SHADOWGRAMS © is a term I have created as an alternative to the traditional term — TANGRAMS.

Tangrams originated in Imperial China during the Tang Dynasty, they are thought to have travelled to Europe in the 19th century on trading ships, and became very popular in Western countries during the WW1.

A **SHADOWGRAM** is a two-dimensional re-arrangement puzzle created by cutting a square into seven pieces. The pieces are actually cut from one large square (See the template on the next page). Here's what you get as you cut out the pieces.

- 2 large right triangles
- 1 medium-sized right triangle
- 2 small right triangles
- 1 small square
- 1 parallelogram

By arranging the seven shapes, they can be fitted together as a large square, rectangle, or triangle. They can also be arranged in a variety of complex shapes, including fanciful ones.

There are many ways to play around with **SHADOWGRAMS** ©. The simplest way is to create your own complex shapes. But traditionally, tangrams are treated as puzzles.

SHADOWGRAMS © can be an individual or partner activity. See pages 6 & 7 for puzzle shapes to create. Solutions to all the puzzles can be found at the back of the book. There are 100's more puzzles on the internet — if you research TANGRAM puzzles.

Large **SHADOWGRAM** © pieces. You can cut out the page from this book and paste it on stiff card or photocopy and laminate.

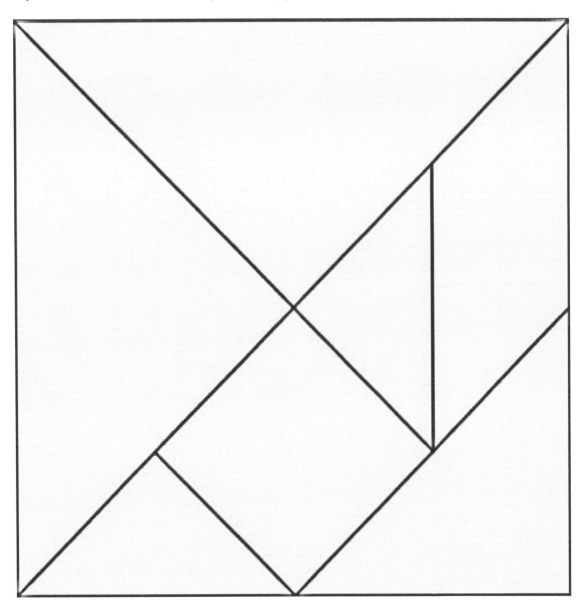

Small SHADOWGRAM © pieces

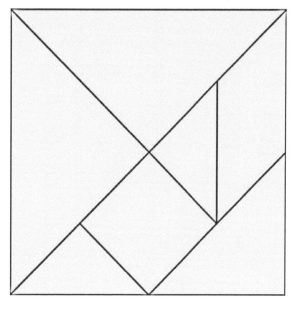

Starter puzzles

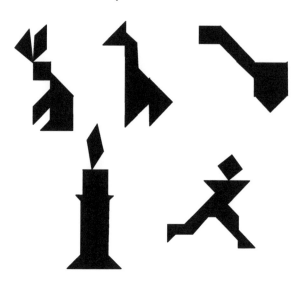

Solutions

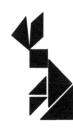 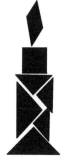 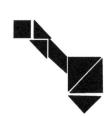 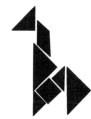 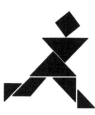

Selection of puzzles to create using you SHADOWGRAM © pieces

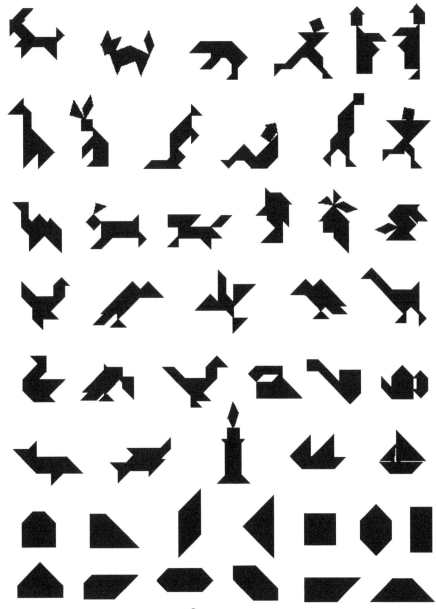

CROSS THE BRIDGE ©

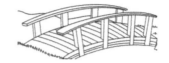

Seven bridges connect five islands. Two of the islands are not connected.

This is a two-player game.

Drawn simply this game looks like this:

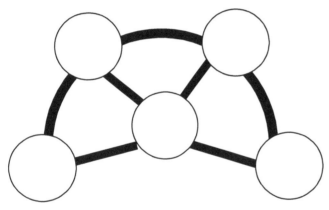

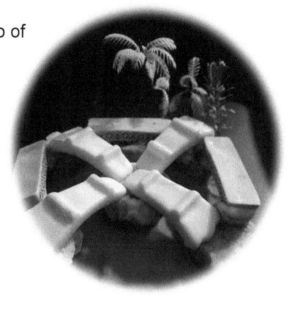

The aim of CROSS THE BRDIGE © is to move one space at a time, to try to trap opponent so that they cannot cross any bridges. (see diag B)

Players take turns to place their markers (use 2 different colored buttons or small pebbles) on the bridge layout … which leaves one bridge unoccupied. (see diag A)

Players can only cross a bridge to a rock island connected by a bridge.

Take turns in moving to an unoccupied (empty) rock island space.

Moving one space at a time, each player attempts to trap their opponent so that they cannot cross any bridges. This is easier said than done … but do not give up. One of the secrets … is to play a fast game.

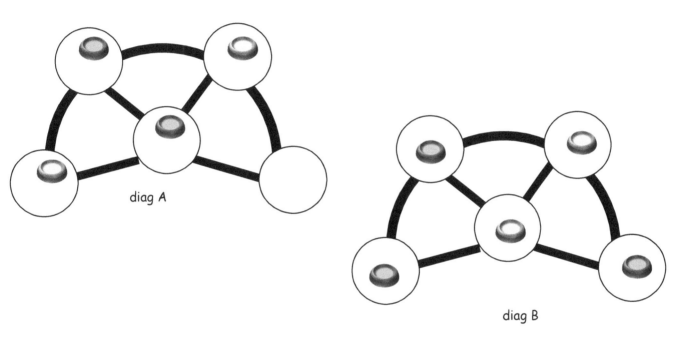

diag A

diag B

The historical origins of this game have been all but lost, apart from the fact that I was using it back in the 1970's with year 5 students as a mathematic extension activity.

You can either use this page or the next to make your playing board.
Cut out or photocopy and laminate.

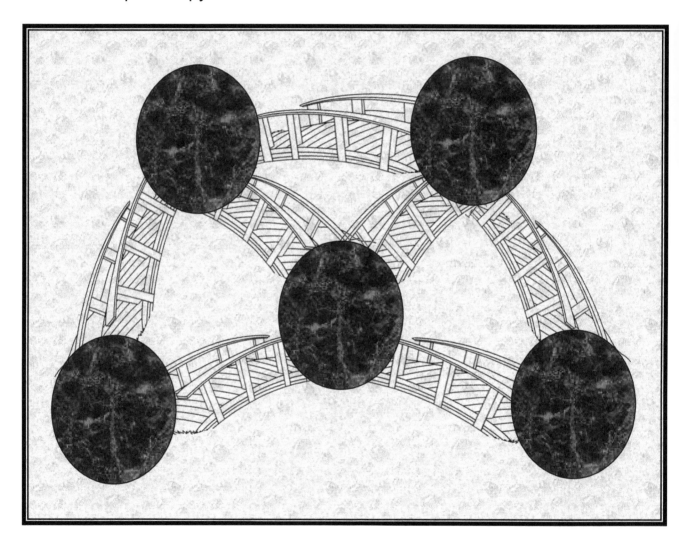

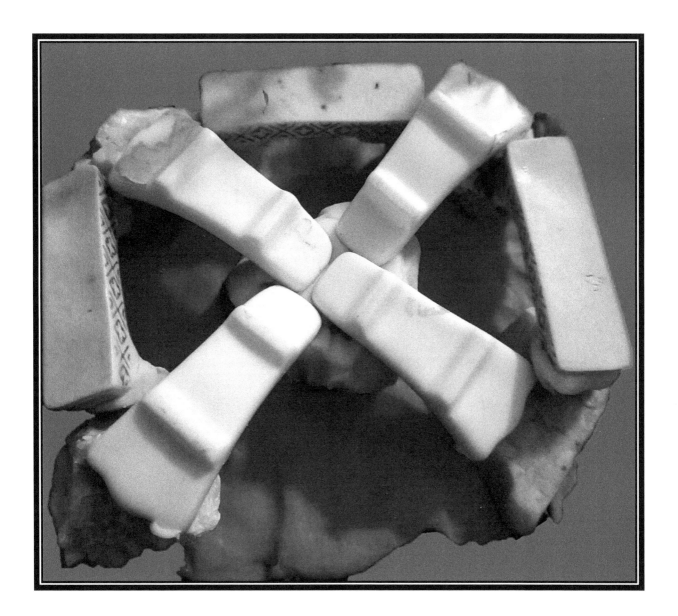

STARCROSS©

AIM OF GAME:

1 PLAYER GAME:

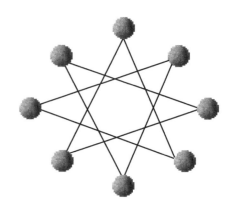

- Try to cover all bases with markers following the correct procedure (see how to play*) or
- To cover as many bases as possible

2 PLAYER GAME:

- To block their opponent by placing the last marker onto one of the bases as players take turns covering bases with markers following the correct procedure*.

*HOW TO PLAY:

If 2 players – take turns. Otherwise play starts anywhere – as they are all empty bases to begin with. Player starts by holding one their markers on empty / unoccupied base and travels across to another empty / unoccupied base along the joining line. They leave their marker there, which means that that base is no longer empty but now occupied.

If 2 players THEN next player – otherwise single player moves to a new empty / unoccupied base and repeats the same procedure of walking and placing marker down to occupy that base.

Play continues in this way until there are no further empty / unoccupied bases available to travel to.

Use the template on the next page, either by cutting out or photocopy and laminate.

You will also need 8 buttons or markers such as small smooth flat beads or pebbles. Diag. C shows the start of play but not the solution. The solution is not given in this book, however through trial and error when you achieve a 7-point game solution … the final piece is simply placed on the last unoccupied space. Players score points as to how many spaces they can cover before being block. In a 2-player game, the player who places the last marker on the STARCROSS layout scores the number of spaces locked.

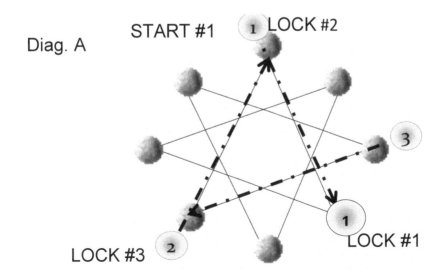

Diag. A

START #1   LOCK #2

LOCK #3   LOCK #1

After the first three moves above, the puzzle would look like this:

Diag. B

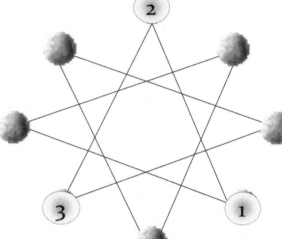

However, a locked-out game would look like this, and in this case would score 5 points, as there are no unoccupied spaces left to move to.

Diag. C

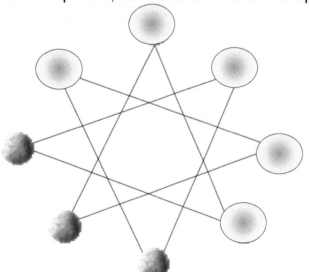

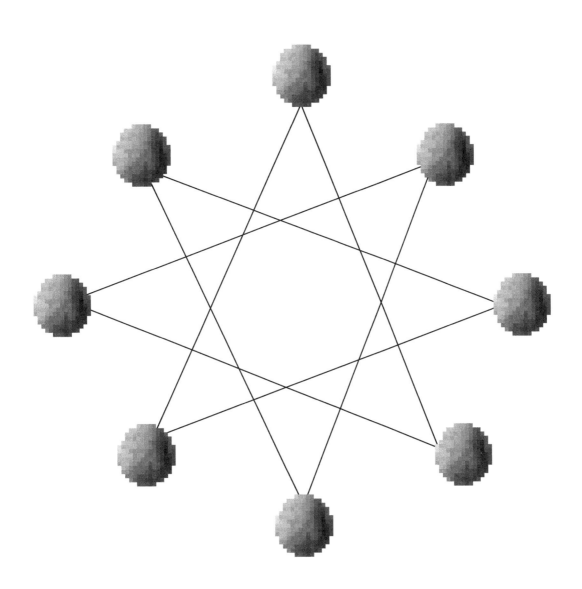

KONO: *4 IN A ROW*

- ◆ 4 X 4 grid (see diag. B)
- ◆ 2 player
- ◆ 4 markers 2 x 2 colours

Historically **KONO: *4 IN A ROW*** is a simplified version of Four Field Kono — an ancient traditional Korean strategy game.

Set up the board as shown in diag. A on the next page.

* To be WINNER …aim to line up your 'MARKERS' anywhere on the board — *HORIZONTALLY OR VERTICALLY* — 4 in a row

* *Diagonal* MOVES **NOT ALLOWED**.

* Move one square at a time. Horizontally or vertically

* No jumping … only one MARKER — one a space at a time. And there is no capturing or taking off an opponent's marker from the board.

A player can only win horizontally or vertically.

On page 18 you can cut out or photocopy and laminate the blank template.

Diag. A

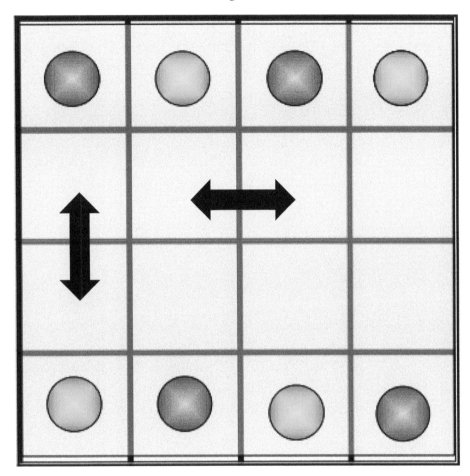

Diag. B

ARROWDOKU©

A pictorial (non-numeric) variation of Sudoku.

AIM: to set each of the arrows in the grid (using the same grid layout - diag. B on page 18) with each arrow facing a different direction in each row and column but not diagonally. ←→↑↓

Use the arrow stencil below — either cut out from this page or photocopy and laminate.

You could also use a soft rubber-foam fabric to cut out the arrows.

- Level one — just use one colour
- Level two — use 4 colours. No colours the same in any row or column. And the arrows must be facing different directions.
- Advanced levels: try using different shapes such as letters e.g. 'L' or 'T' or coloured buttons.

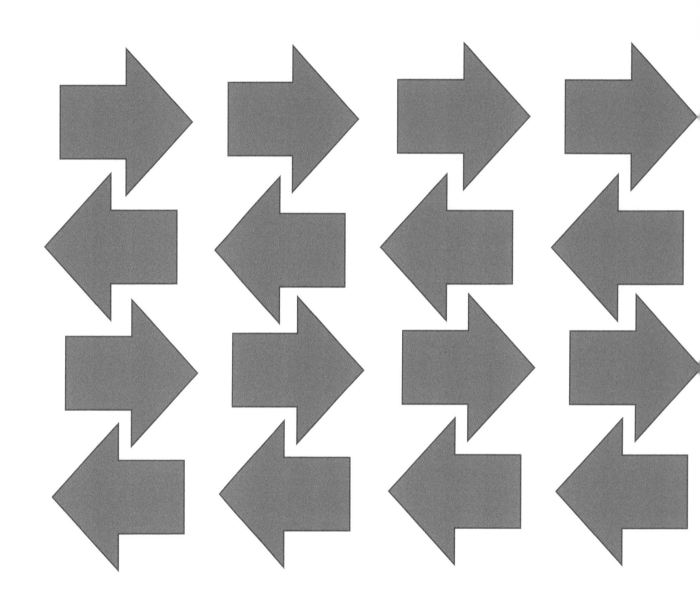

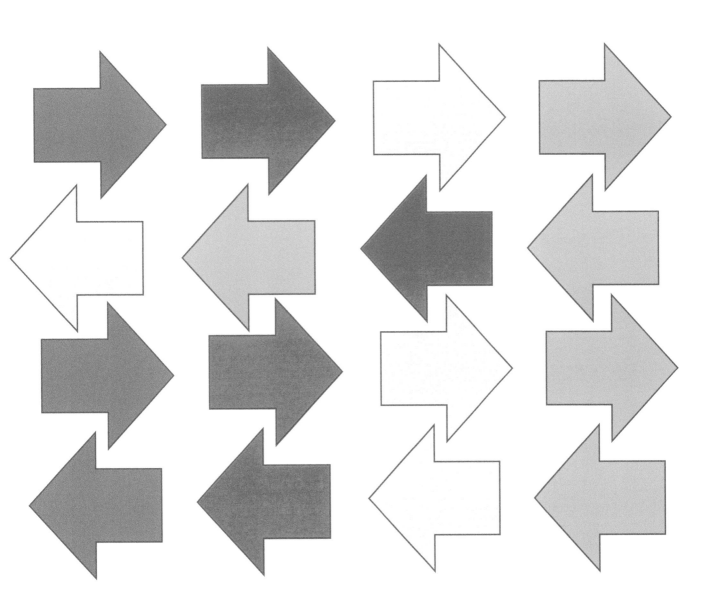

MAGIC SQUARES

MAGIC SQUARES is a non-numerical variation of the popular '15 puzzle' (also called Gem Puzzle, Boss Puzzle, Game of Fifteen, Mystic Square and many others) dating back to 1874.

This can be either a single person or a partner puzzle activity.

AIM OF GAME:

To manoeuvre the markers around the grid one space at a time— vertically & horizontally to solve the PUZZLE MAP. (see diag. A on page 23)

MATERIALS REQUIRED:

- PUZZLE MAPS (see diags. #1 - #9—page 25)
- Cut out or photocopy your set of PUZZLE MAPS (laminate)
- 8 markers required — 2 x 4 colours.
- Use buttons or plastic discs or similar
- For 3 x 3 grid use the grid on page 24. Cut out or photocopy and laminate.
- For a 4 x 4 grid — same as for ARROWDUKO & KONO

LAYOUT:

3 x 3 grid

Shuffle and turn face down your PUZZLE MAP cards. Place your coloured markers randomly onto grid. Turn over the top PUZZLE MAP card and begin to solve the puzzle.

Moving one space at a time into the empty space created each time — horizontally, vertically or diagonally.

No jumps or swapping around of markers

Continue until the puzzle is solved.

NOTE: *every PUZZLE MAP is solvable.*

ADVANCED PLAY—4 x 4 grid

For the ambitious!!! Set up a 4 x 4 grid. Create your own new set of PUZZLE MAPS.

Players only move horizontally or vertically.

Players cannot move diagonally or jump or switch markers around.

Other adaptations:

Use 4 or 6 coloured markers.

Using discs numbered from 1 to 15 re-creates a large version of the traditional slotted magic number puzzle.

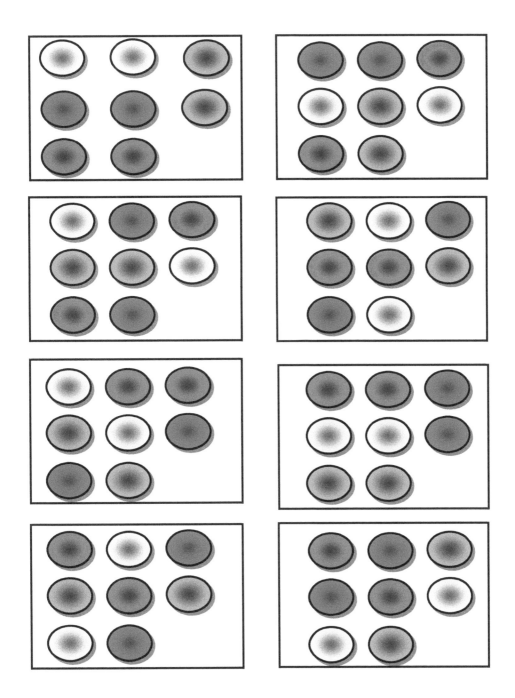

DOMINOE DICE ELIMINATION ©

A game for 1 or 2 players

AIM OF GAME:

To cover as many dominoes as possible with one of your markers, by rolling dice and adding or subtracting numbers shown. <u>Winner</u> has the most number of markers down or disposes of all their markers in the time limit set at the start.

MATERIALS REQUIRED:

- 28 x dominoes

Each with a different total from 1 to 12 e.g.

'1' = 0/1; '2' = 0/2 or 1/1; '3' = 0/3 or 1/2;

'4' = 0/4 or 1/3 or 2/2 ... etc up to '12' = 6/6

- 28 markers
  2 players 14 x 2 colour markers
  Single player — 28 markers any colour
- A pair of dice
- Optional digital-egg timer.

HOW TO PLAY:

Turn all the dominoes face up and spread them out.

Decide who goes first. Player rolls dice.

Then they add or subtract the numbers to get a score for example

This would give a score of 7 if added or 5 if subtracted.

The player would then place one of their markers onto the domino showing either a total 5 or 7. *NOTE*: 5 domino should be a 5-dot end and a blank dot end. It could also be a 4 &1, or 3 & 2 combo .Whereas the 7 domino could be 4 & 3, 5 & 2 or 6 & 1. Once a domino is 'marked' then it is turn upside down with that player's coloured marked on top.

If their domino score has been covered with a marker already, then you can quickly re-calculate before the next person has their turn, and look for another domino. If you discover no domino is available then in a single-player game, this would mean a loss of a point scored. For a 2-player game you forfeit being able to place a marker for that turn.

In a 2-player game, throwing a double dice score allows the player to have a bonus turn—regardless of whether they have placed a marker or not.

If time runs out because of certain combinations not being rolled as in 6 & 6; make sure that you give every player sufficient warning about finishing e.g. "2 rolls left for everyone."

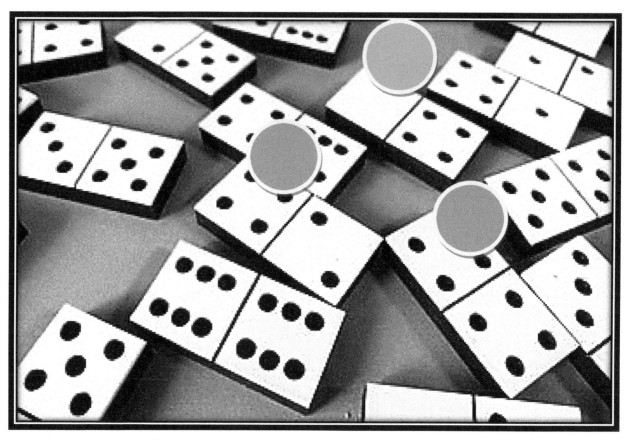

Advance playing: players could also multiply or divide the numbers thrown on the dice as well as adding or subtracting.

FIVE FIELD KONO

This is a traditional Korean game. In English it is known as Five Field Kono. In Korean, it is called *"O-PAT-KO-NO"*. It was first recorded in the west in 1895.

AIM OF GAME:

To move all of your *MEN* to the opposite side of the board first — by only moving **DIAGONALLY**.

MATERIALS REQUIRED:

- 4 x 4 grid (same as for ARROWDOKU & KONO)
- The points of the grid create the playing field rather than the spaces (see diag. #1)
- 14 markers
    - 7 x 2 colour markers

- grid as shown (see diag. #1)

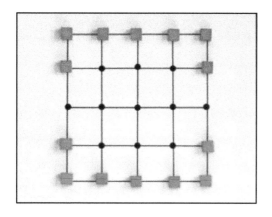

Diag. #1 Starting positions

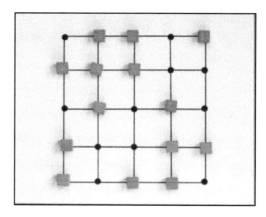

Diag. #2 Game in play

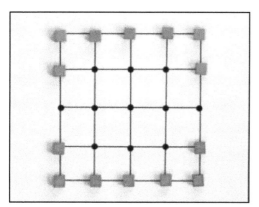

Diag. #3 Finishing positions

HOW TO PLAY:

Set up the board as shown in diag. #1

* Players move <u>one grid-point at a time</u> ... *only diagonally*

* Players can move forwards and backwards diagonally

* **No horizontal or vertical moves**

* A variation to the traditional rules:

>   *JUMPING is PERMITTED ... but not until you have at least 2 MEN 'home'.*

31

❖ Diagonal jumps only – over any coloured marker
❖ No capturing of opponent's MEN
* Only one *MAN* in each grid-space at a time

* REMEMBER: *YOU CAN ONLY WIN BY GETTING ALL YOUR MEN ONTO THE OTHER SIDE OF BOARD IN THE SAME PATTERN.*

As an alternative to using the points of a 4 x 4 grid. You could use the spaces of a 5 x 5 grid, moving diagonally across the spaces, as shown in diag. #4

diag. #4

AROUND THE MILL©

Traditionally known as Nine Men's Morris

A two-person game

HISTORY

The oldest recording of this game is on a building with the board layout carved into its stones — an temple at Kurna, Egypt, which dating roughly about 1400 BCE. However, it is not known when the game board itself was engraved.

There are many Nine Men's Morris carved into various buildings' stones throughout the Roman Empire and in the seats of many medieval cathedrals.

This game is known by many names, such as Mill or Windmill, most probably, because the shape of the board looks somewhat like a windmill, and Merrels, from the Latin word *merellus,* which means "gaming piece".

The name Nine Men's Morris seems to have been originated by Shakespeare in his play, A Midsummer Night's Dream (Act II, Scene I), in which Titania refers to such a board by saying, "The nine men's morris is filled up with mud".

Equipment

The game of **AROUND THE MILL**© is played on a board consisting of three concentric squares connected by lines from the middle of each of the inner square's sides to the middle of the corresponding outer square's side. See Diag. #2 on page 36.

Pieces are played on the corner points and on the points where lines intersect so there are 24 playable points. Each player will have 9 marker-pieces called 'Men'. Different colours for each player.

Preparation and Objective

The basic aim of Nine Mens Morris is to make "mills" – as in vertical or horizontal lines of **three in a row**. Every time this is achieved, an opponent's piece is removed, the overall objective being to reduce the number of opponent's pieces to less than three or to render the opponent unable to play. At the start, the board is empty.

Basic Play

Players decide who will play the light colour — as the light colour moves first and has a slight advantage as a result. Play is in two phases.

> PHASE ONE: To begin with, players take turns to play a piece of their own colour on any unoccupied point until all eighteen pieces have been played.
>
> PHASE TWO: Play continues alternately by each player moving one piece along a line to an adjacent point.
>
> During both of these phases, whenever a player achieves a mill, that player immediately **removes** from the board **one piece** belonging to the opponent that **does not form part of a mill.**

It is only upon the formation of a mill that a piece is captured. A player can break their own mill by moving a piece out of it and then, in a subsequent turn, play the piece back again, thus forming a new mill and capturing another piece.

Captured pieces are never replayed onto the board and remain captured for the remainder of the game. The game is finished when a player loses either by being reduced to two pieces or by being unable to move. See Diag. #1

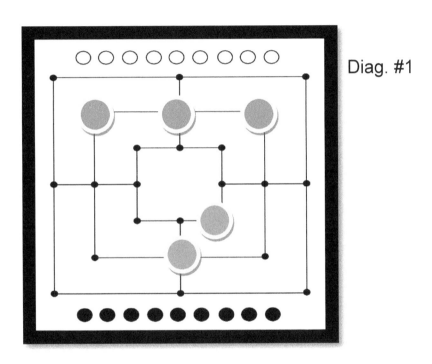

Diag. #1

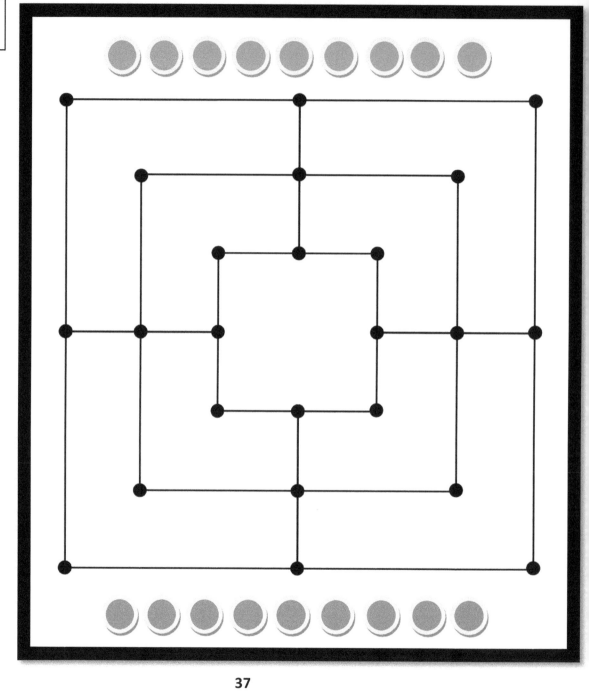

NIM: TREASURE

Variants of Nim have been played since ancient times. The game is said to have originated in China—it closely resembles the Chinese game of 捡石子 *jiǎn-shízi*, or "picking stones"—but the origin is uncertain. The earliest European references to Nim are from the beginning of the 16th century. Its current name was coined by Charles L. Bouton of Harvard University, who also developed the complete theory of the game in 1901, but the origins of the name were never fully explained.

There are various ways to play Nim — a strategy game for two players.

The game can also be played in 3 piles of 3 – 5 – 7 counters / discs / coins (15 total).

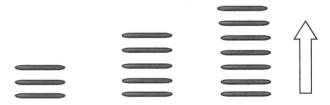

Discs / counter / coins can be removed either 1, 2 or 3 at a time. Player left with the last disc is the loser. In other words, to be the winner you must attempt to leave the last disc for your opponent.

Sticks, shells or small pebbles can also be used arranged in lines.

NOTE: **NIM: TREASURE** specifically identifies one piece as the TREASURE to be the last piece.

On the next two pages are a couple of layout variations.

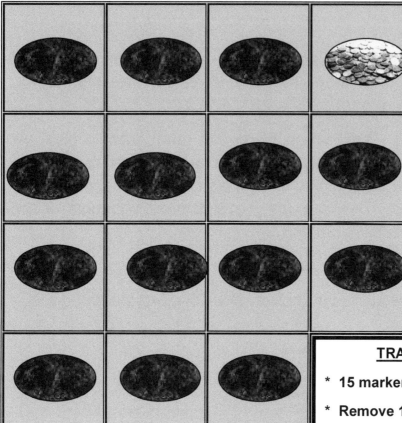

Using these layouts does not require a printout of a board. Just use the layout suggestions as shown with the markers.

TRADTIONAL RULES

* **15 markers —one on each square.**

* **Remove 1, 2 or 3 marker at a time**

* **Aim to be the *WINNER* ... leave one marker**

* **Player left with one pot / marker — *LOSES*.**

TREASURE RULES

- **Player who is left with TREASURE wins**
- **TREASURE can be placed anywhere**

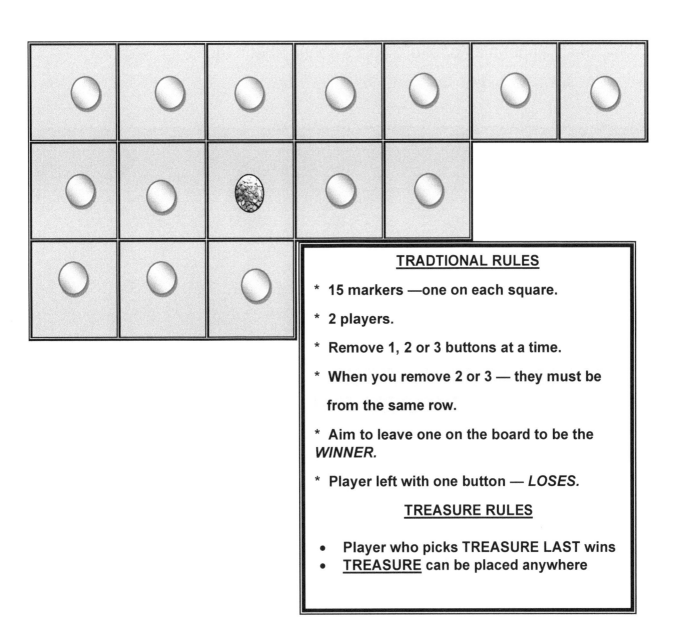

TRADTIONAL RULES

* 15 markers —one on each square.

* 2 players.

* Remove 1, 2 or 3 buttons at a time.

* When you remove 2 or 3 — they must be

   from the same row.

* Aim to leave one on the board to be the *WINNER.*

* Player left with one button — *LOSES.*

TREASURE RULES

• Player who picks TREASURE LAST wins
• <u>TREASURE</u> can be placed anywhere

Use of small pebbles or shells offers a kinesthetic-tactile experience.

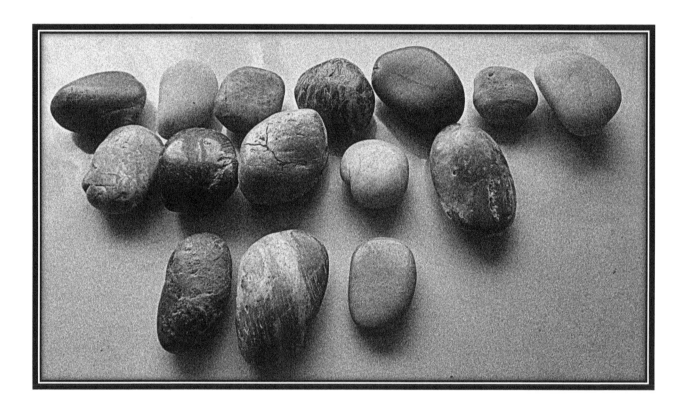

APPENDIX

➢ The following pages are provided for those who do not want to remove pages from the middle of the book. These pages can be removed for laminating. Lamination is the best way to preserve the playing boards.

➢ Markers or playing pieces can be made from cardboard, plastic discs, other board game pieces such as checkers, coins, buttons, small pebbles or shells.

➢ The last page is the solutions page for SHADOWGRAMS©

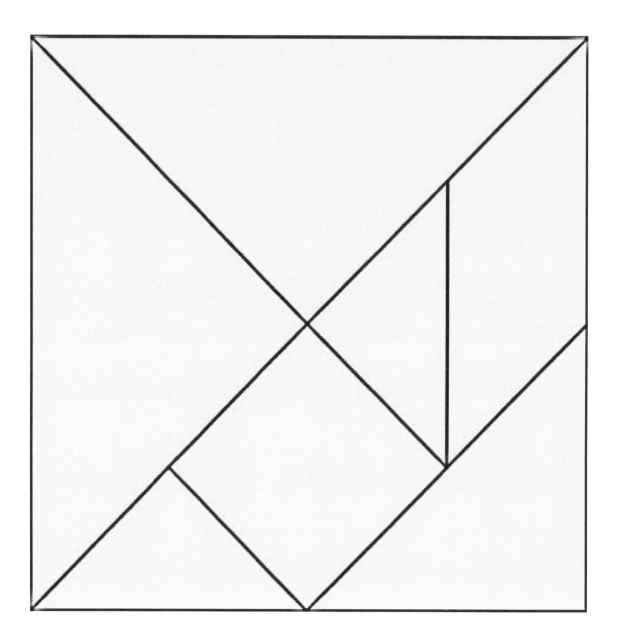

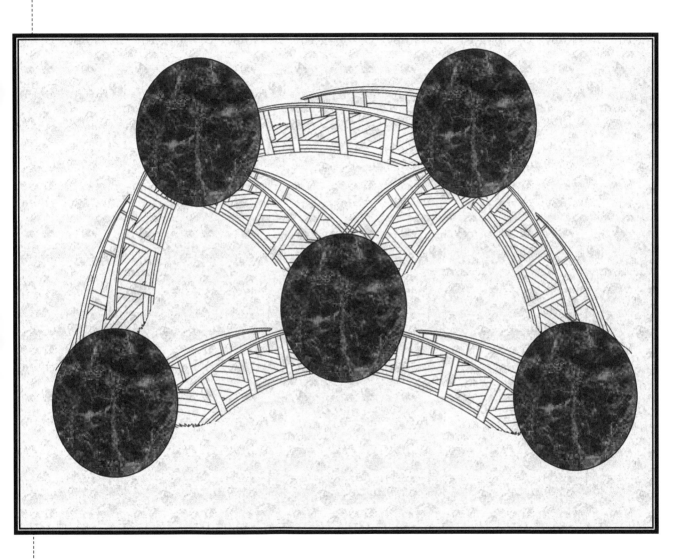

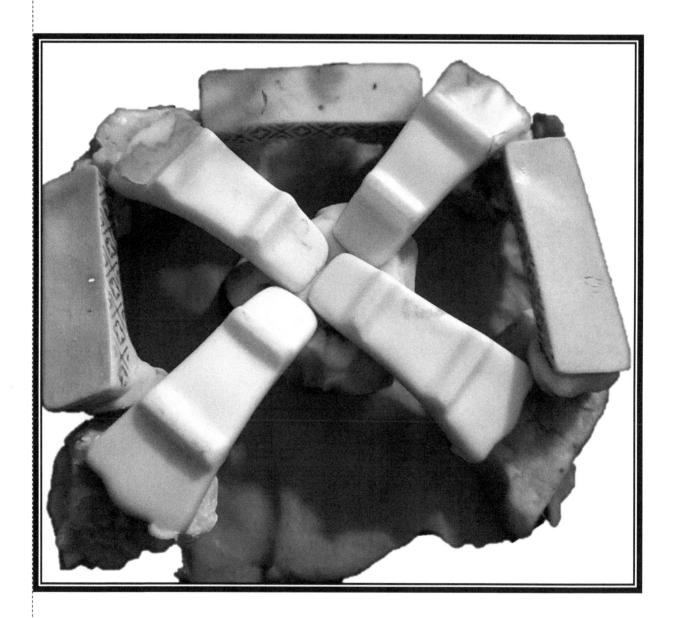

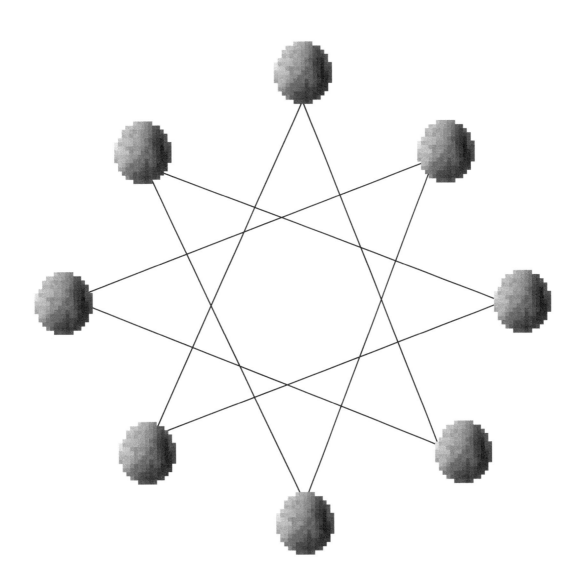

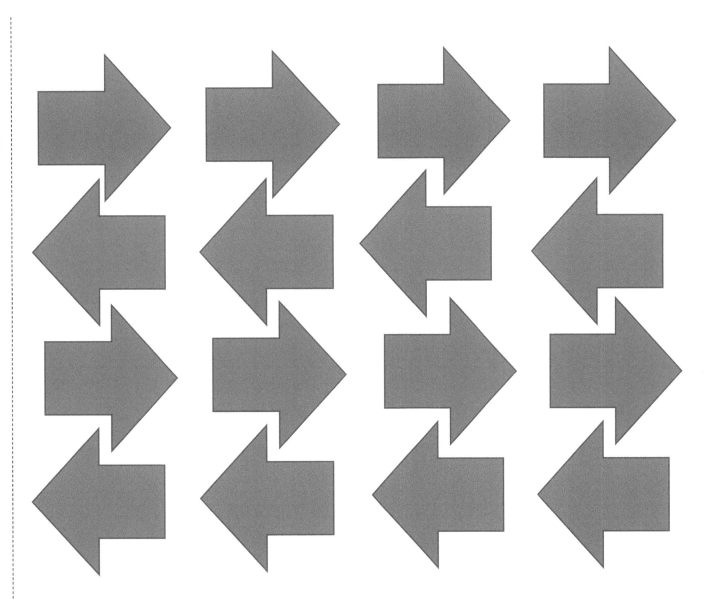

48

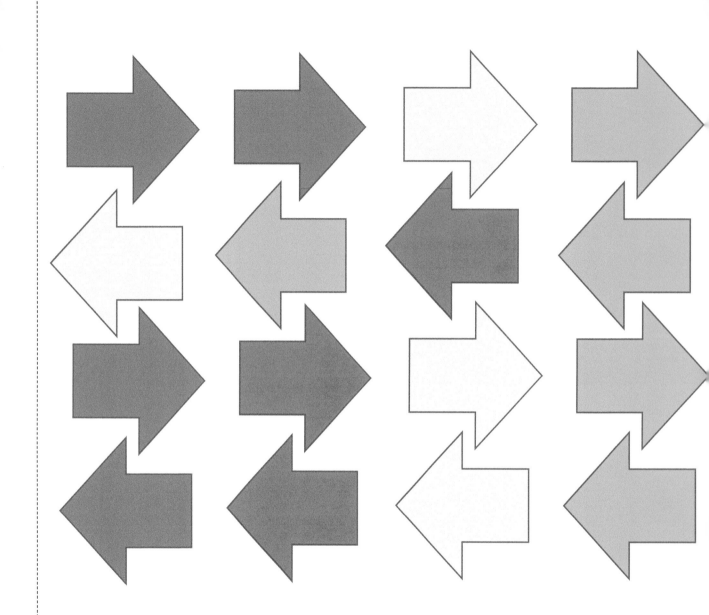

49

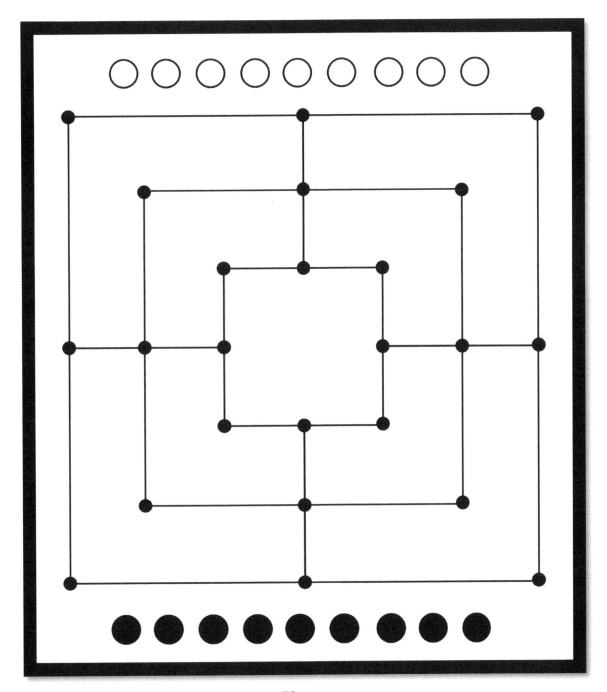

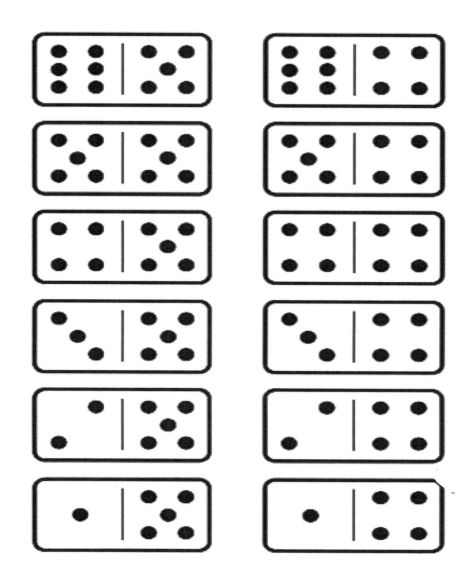

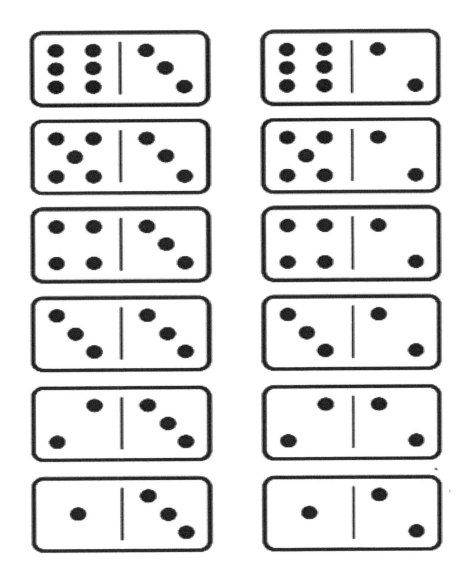

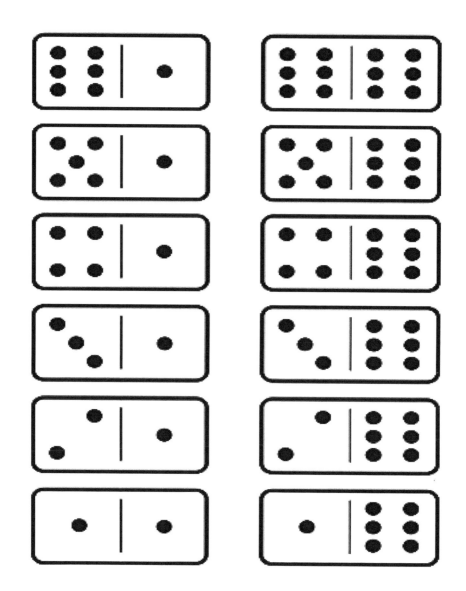

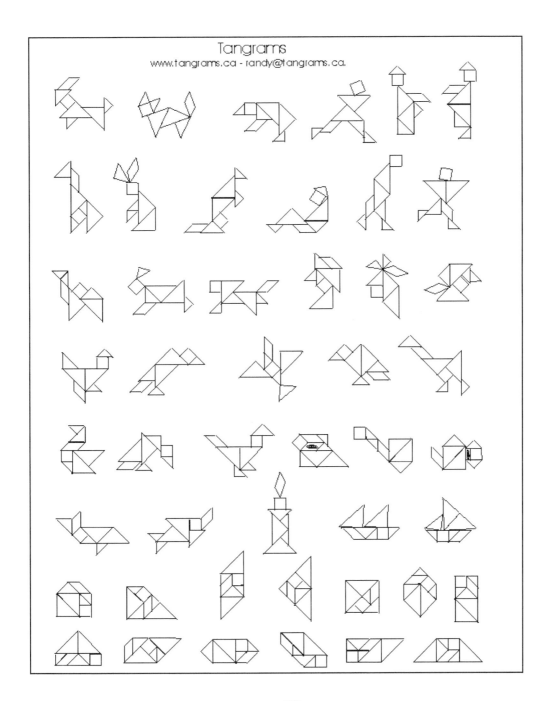

Lightning Source UK Ltd.
Milton Keynes UK
UKHW051032050123
414827UK00004B/109